MW01223008

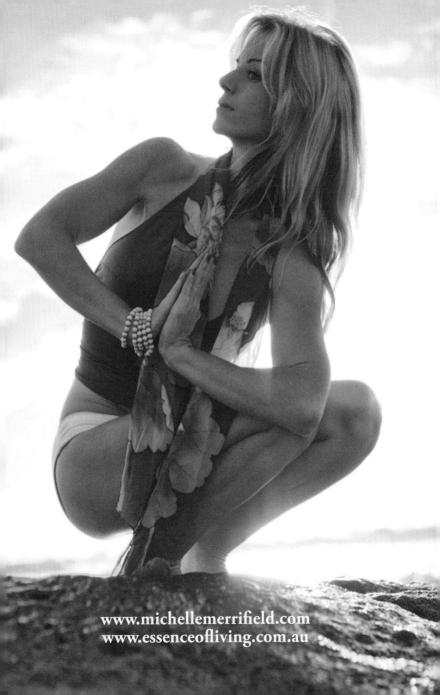

www.michellemerrifield.com
www.essenceofliving.com.au

First printed 2012.

Copyright Michelle Merrifield.
www.michellemerrifield.com

Designed by Michelle Merrifield.
Edited by Michelle Merrifield and Mel Brady.

Images © 2013 Gary Howard, Alana in Love,
shutterstock.com, istockphoto.com.

While every effort has been made to acknowledge the author of the
quotations used, please notify the publisher if this has not occurred.

Designed with love in Australia.

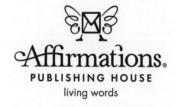

Affirmations.
PUBLISHING HOUSE
living words

author's note

I would like to express my gratitude and appreciation by dedicating this book to those who without you in my life, nothing would be possible. To my beautiful sister who is the light of life, to the students I have met since starting my business, my amazing angels working at Essence of Living, my beloved partner, and my puppies.

buddhaful

(boo-duh-fuhl); adjective.

A reference used to describe someone or something that embodies a Buddha like nature and beautiful attributes inside and out.

contents

manifesto

As a Body Buddhaful I, _____ promise to:

- ◆ **dream** and **create** a vision for my future
- ◆ know I can **change the world**
- ◆ build **loving relationships** with friends and family
- ◆ practice **peace** at home
- ◆ practice **mindfulness** and **positivity**
- ◆ exercise for **fun** daily
- ◆ create a **sacred** space to nourish my **soul** at home and work
- ◆ **challenge** myself daily
- ◆ **love** my body
- ◆ **face** my fears
- ◆ **empty the trash** from my mind and let go of emotions
- ◆ schedule daily **herbal tea** sipping and **journal** writing
- ◆ be **generous** and **grateful**
- ◆ **nourish my spirit** with singing, dancing and music
- ◆ connect with **nature**
- ◆ **love animals** big and small
- ◆ sleep soundly at night with a **light heart**
- ◆ **breathe** through challenges
- ◆ practice **Ethical Eating**
- ◆ surround myself with inspiring people and **be inspired**
- ◆ **inspire** others
- ◆ nourish my body with water, **fresh fruit** and **vegetables**
- ◆ travel and **explore** the wonders of the world
- ◆ practice **self-discipline** and a good work ethic
- ◆ continue to read, learn and **grow**

Signature _____ Date _____

how to use me

Within the pages of this buddhaful journal, you are given the opportunity to look within and discover yourself on a deeper level. The journaling is repetitive in nature, answering the same friendly yet confronting questions week to week. Similar to the ocean constantly moving in waves; so are our feelings, thoughts, perspectives and priorities always changing like the tide across the seashore. Each week the same question will appear taking you deeper into the vast ocean that is your spirit, guiding you the same way a compass guides a sailor, helping you find your truth. The simple act of writing is therapeutic in nature; it helps us become clear and honest with ourselves.

Remember this is YOUR journal therefore precious, so treat it with love and respect, like you would an old friend. Each time you put pen to pad, be mindful of the power of words; write everything your heart desires, including those thoughts you have trouble giving a voice. This journal has the ability to shape and transform your life.

Before you begin journaling, create a sacred space, light a candle, play your favourite music, pour a cup of tea, turn off your phone and breathe deeply to centre your mind and connect with your spirit. Sit still for at least 5 minutes meditating on the day's enquiry, allowing it to move through your mind, body and spirit before answering. You will be amazed what may come up if you give yourself some time to process your thoughts and feelings.

There will be good and bad days just like there are sunny and rainy days. Neither can be viewed as better than the other as it's all a part of life. Just write in the moment and go beyond the weather of your emotions. Don't be afraid to challenge yourself, going deeper beyond your comfort zone as this is where the magic happens.

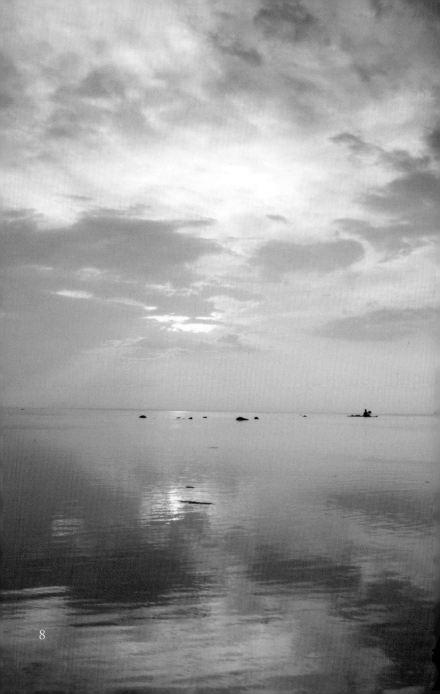

goal setting

The most important aspect in goal setting is ensuring there is a strong emotional driver along with a burning desire for your goal. The whole reason we haven't achieved our goals to date is because they often require sacrifice and massive action for realisation.

We can all dream about how we want our lives to unfold. The hard part is actually fine tuning the details of how that actually looks, feels, tastes, sounds and smells. This is how you need to write your goals. Write a relevant, realistic and time-bound goal. One in which you can see yourself manifesting this experience., i.e. I will run 10 kilometres by the 1st of September.

Once you have a sense of how it feels to be in your future achieving your goals, you can work backwards on how to get there. What courses, negotiations, conversations, commitments and sacrifices are needed in order for your dreams to come true? You will need to build a comprehensive action plan.

If your goal is to lose 5 kilograms within 5 weeks, what will you have to stop eating and start doing in order to achieve that goal week-to-week, day-to-day? Most people don't go into depth with their detail and that's why most people don't achieve their goals. We won't let this happen: A good solid plan will help you achieve and succeed in your goals.

Once you have completed your action plan, you will begin the most challenging part of achieving your goals... following through with your plan!

In the words of the Dalai Lama, **"judge your success by what you had to give up in order to get it."** Self-discipline and a positive mental attitude are essential for success. Surround yourself with people who inspire you and will support you when times get tough. Your circle of friends can really influence your outcomes.

be still & breathe

Meditation is an alluring art many seek to learn yet can be very difficult to master. The first element to explore is finding the space where you want to begin your meditation practice. Find yourself a comfortable and cozy area where you can sit with minimal distractions. This is not as easy as it sounds as there will always be distractions surrounding you: The bird will sing too loud, the wind will blow too hard and the dog up the road will start barking. Finding contentment whilst being surrounded by these challenges is all part of the process of accepting the things you are unable to change and learning to ease into the never-ending noise that surrounds you.

Once you have found the quietest place in your home, ensure it is warm, welcoming and clutter free. You may even wish to decorate the area with candles, flowers and pictures of those you love. It helps if you develop a regular routine where you can sit and be still. By having this familiar time and location you will begin to build a positive vibration and over time you will notice the moment you sit down, you will instantly begin to relax and soften physically and mentally allowing you to drop into stillness.

Now it's time to sit and check in with your body, so prop yourself up on a blanket, cushion or bolster for support and begin to settle into your seat. Make sure your knees are lower than your hips allowing your pelvis to anteriorly tilt, your heart to open and your spine to lengthen. Make sure you are comfortable as you will be in this position for a while. Start with 5 minutes of meditation daily and eventually progress to 20 minutes each day.

Once you have found your sacred space; commit to it, be still and resist the urge and temptation to move or fidget. Shift your focus to your breath, making sure you are breathing in and out through your nose. Start to notice how your breath affects your body, the cool air that rolls into the nostrils and the warm air that leaves the nostrils. Feel it rush down your throat as your whole body relaxes, deepening with each breath. You will notice the better your posture, the better the quality of your breath.

There are four parts to the complete yogic breath; the breath should reach the belly, side body, back and chest. This will maximise your breathing capacity aiming to breathe in for the count of four and out for the count of four. Inhale into each body part starting at the belly and finishing at the chest and each exhale releasing the air in reverse, starting with the chest and emptying the belly last. This in itself will induce a meditative state. By focusing on the directional movement of the breath in the body, it will help to clear your mind.

As you relax into your breath begin to extend the duration of the breath to a count of 5, 6, 7, 8, 9 or 10 ensuring the inhalation and exhalation are practiced equally. Be mindful not to strain or cause discomfort during this practice as the aim isn't about stretching the breath, it's about stretching your mind into stillness. Continue to develop your practice and all will be revealed…

~ the better your posture, the better the quality of your breath.

eat with love

Eating should be seen as a joyful experience and the opportunity to nourish and feed your temple, the house of your spirit. We have lost the art of eating and making food with love. Food is something that should be enjoyed, savoured and shared with those you love. The ritual of eating has been celebrated for as long as mankind has been on planet earth. Eating and great festivity shared with friends and family go hand in hand.

Eating itself is not the problem we face, we need to eat to survive. It is what we are eating and how much of it that we need to be mindful of. One of the best ways to start taking control of your health is learning the wonderful art of cooking. This way you can be completely aware of what goes into the food you make and avoid the risk of consuming toxic chemicals and additives found in packaged foods. You will soon learn how much sugar, salt and fat goes into different dishes and be able to understand which foods are healthier than others.

There is a deep connection with our ancient ancestors that cooking from scratch creates. Knowing that you are using organic natural ingredients filled with energy and vitality, mixed with home grown herbs, added with a pinch of creativity and a dollop of faith, prepared with love and served with a smile gives a feeling of harmony and contentment.

Eat from the earth what is whole and natural, listen to your body and feel how different foods affect your energy, mood and weight. Experiment and enjoy a wide variety of different fruits and vegetables, eat in season and always support your local farmer by buying fresh produce. Plant herb gardens and learn how to sprout. Be creative and try a new recipe as often as you can even if it's simply a new juice blend to keep food fun and interesting. Share your masterpieces with friends and family and enjoy the art of ethical eating.

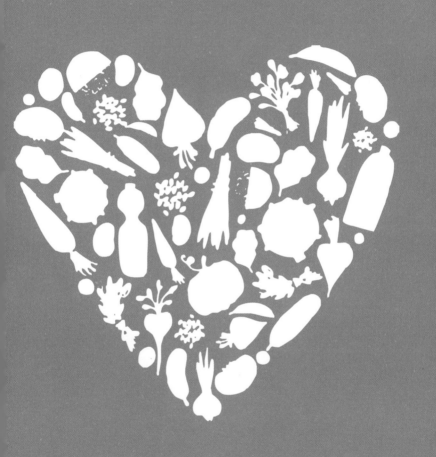

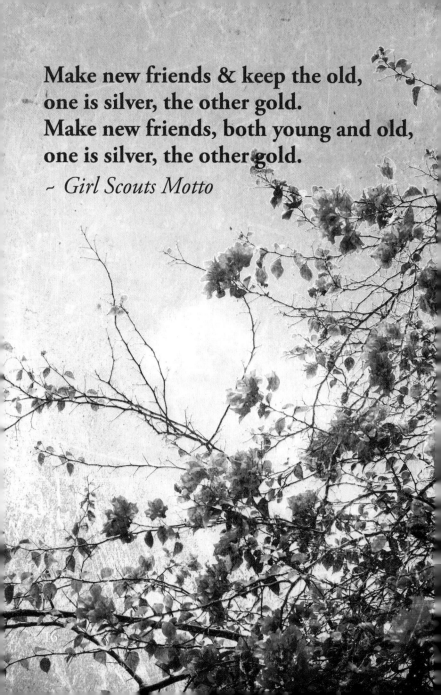

Make new friends & keep the old,
one is silver, the other gold.
Make new friends, both young and old,
one is silver, the other gold.

~ *Girl Scouts Motto*

vision board

write your favourite friendship quote
stick a photo of you & your friends here

week one

What exercises have I completed and for what duration?
How have my energy levels and moods been affected today?

_____

_____

_____

_____

_____

_____

_____

_____

What foods and portion sizes have I eaten today?
How have my energy levels and moods been affected today?

_____

_____

_____

_____

_____

_____

day one

I am grateful for

week one

What exercises have I completed and for what duration?
How have my energy levels and moods been affected today?

_____

_____

_____

_____

_____

_____

_____

_____

What foods and portion sizes have I eaten today?
How have my energy levels and moods been affected today?

_____

_____

_____

_____

_____

_____

day two

I am ready to let go of _____

week one

What exercises have I completed and for what duration?
How have my energy levels and moods been affected today?

What foods and portion sizes have I eaten today?
How have my energy levels and moods been affected today?

----

day three

I love my body because _____

_____

_____

_____

_____

_____

_____

_____

_____

_____

_____

_____

_____

_____

_____

_____

_____

_____

_____

_____

_____

_____

walking with friends

From your very first step as a young child, to walking into your first day at school or walking home after a big day of work, walking is the link that threads our lives and experiences together. Each step filled with memories leads us to where we are today. Over the years we have shared our journey with our friends and family and what better way to spend quality time than to share a walk.

Walking is a wonderful easy low-impact exercise filled with health benefits and what better way to reap these benefits than whilst connecting and conversing with those we love. This camaraderie encourages conversation and motivation as you share your daily highs and lows along the path of life. Walking is not only good for the heart but also for matters of the heart. You can learn about each other, help one another with life's challenges, grow together and maintain your health together. There's nothing like this kind of camaraderie to inspire and put a little life in your step.

Walking promotes feelings of pleasure, tranquility and well-being, and helps relieve the pain of depression by encouraging the production of the body's natural opiates called endorphins. Habitual walkers also benefit from increased energy levels, greater stamina and a sounder sleep at night.

So find a friend and begin your walking programme today. When in doubt, I'm sure you can find a four-legged furry friend that would love to go for a walk with you.

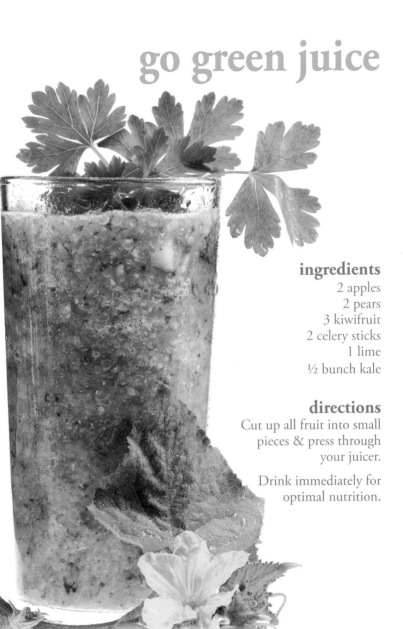

go green juice

ingredients
2 apples
2 pears
3 kiwifruit
2 celery sticks
1 lime
½ bunch kale

directions
Cut up all fruit into small
pieces & press through
your juicer.

Drink immediately for
optimal nutrition.

week one

What exercises have I completed and for what duration?
How have my energy levels and moods been affected today?

_____

_____

_____

_____

_____

_____

_____

_____

What foods and portion sizes have I eaten today?
How have my energy levels and moods been affected today?

_____

_____

_____

_____

_____

_____

day four

I am fearful of _____

_____

_____

_____

_____

_____

_____

_____

_____

_____

_____

_____

_____

_____

_____

_____

_____

_____

week one

What exercises have I completed and for what duration?
How have my energy levels and moods been affected today?

What foods and portion sizes have I eaten today?
How have my energy levels and moods been affected today?

----

day five

My dreams and plans are

week one

What exercises have I completed and for what duration?
How have my energy levels and moods been affected today?

What foods and portion sizes have I eaten today?
How have my energy levels and moods been affected today?

----

day six

Today I made someone happy because

week one

What exercises have I completed and for what duration?
How have my energy levels and moods been affected today?

What foods and portion sizes have I eaten today?
How have my energy levels and moods been affected today?

----

day seven

I will change the world by ....

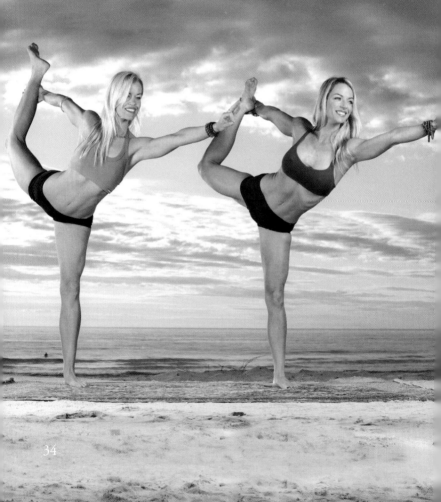

"What can you do to
promote world peace?
Go home and love your family."
~ Mother Teresa

34

vision board

write your favourite family quote
stick a photo of you & your family here

week two

What exercises have I completed and for what duration?
How have my energy levels and moods been affected today?

What foods and portion sizes have I eaten today?
How have my energy levels and moods been affected today?

----

day one

I am grateful for ....

week two

What exercises have I completed and for what duration?
How have my energy levels and moods been affected today?

What foods and portion sizes have I eaten today?
How have my energy levels and moods been affected today?

I am ready to let go of

week two

What exercises have I completed and for what duration?
How have my energy levels and moods been affected today?

What foods and portion sizes have I eaten today?
How have my energy levels and moods been affected today?

I love my body because ....

....

....

....

....

....

....

....

....

....

....

....

....

....

....

....

....

....

....

....

....

swimming

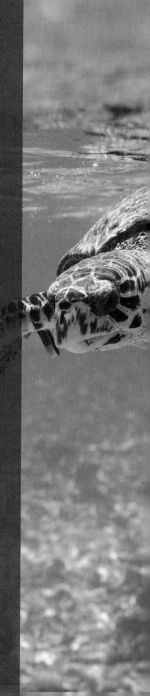

It's no wonder we are attracted to water when the human body is on average 60% water. The brain alone is composed of 70% water, the lungs at nearly 90%, our blood at about 83% and the planet is 70% water, so it's only natural we feel connected and at home in water.

So what better way to connect with nature than swimming in beautiful beaches, rock pools, lakes, dams and rivers and to cool down on a hot summer day? Swimming is a healthy, low-cost, low-impact activity that you can continue throughout your life with numerous physical and mental health benefits. Swimming is a great workout as you move your whole body resisting against water.

Swimming is one of the best forms of exercise for people with asthma as you are less likely to experience asthma symptoms, because when you're swimming, you are breathing in air near the surface of the water that is warmer and more humid (moist) than normal air.

Swimming training can increase the volume of the lungs as well as helping to develop good breathing techniques making this type of exercise is excellent for improving muscle tone and general fitness.

moroccan chickpea & couscous salad

Preparation and cooking time: 20 minutes

ingredients

1 cup quick cooking couscous
¼ cup raisins
½ cup vegetable stock
3 tablespoons extra virgin olive oil
2 tablespoons lemon juice
1 clove garlic – minced
1 teaspoon ground cumin
1 teaspoon ground coriander
1 teaspoon ground ginger
1 teaspoon salt
1 carrot – grated
½ red pepper – finely diced
¼ red onion – finely diced
2 tablespoons chopped flat leaf parsley
1 cup canned chickpeas – rinsed and drained

directions

Mix couscous with raisins in a bowl and add boiling vegetable stock.

Cover with a plate or plastic wrap to seal in the steam and let sit for 5 minutes. Place the oil, lemon juice, garlic, spices and salt in a jar with a screw top lid and shake to mix.

Fluff couscous with a fork to separate the grains and stir through the carrot, red pepper, onion, chickpeas and parsley.

Pour over the dressing and toss together until well combined.

week two

What exercises have I completed and for what duration?
How have my energy levels and moods been affected today?

What foods and portion sizes have I eaten today?
How have my energy levels and moods been affected today?

I am fearful of ....

....

....

....

....

....

....

....

....

....

....

....

....

....

....

....

....

....

....

week two

What exercises have I completed and for what duration?
How have my energy levels and moods been affected today?

What foods and portion sizes have I eaten today?
How have my energy levels and moods been affected today?

----

day five

My dreams and plans are

week two

What exercises have I completed and for what duration?
How have my energy levels and moods been affected today?

What foods and portion sizes have I eaten today?
How have my energy levels and moods been affected today?

----

day six

Today I made someone happy because

week two

What exercises have I completed and for what duration?
How have my energy levels and moods been affected today?

What foods and portion sizes have I eaten today?
How have my energy levels and moods been affected today?

----

day seven

I will change the world by _____

_____

_____

_____

_____

_____

_____

_____

_____

_____

_____

_____

_____

_____

_____

_____

"Humankind has not woven the web of life. We are but one thread within it. Whatever we do to the web, we do to ourselves. All things are bound together. All things connect."

- Chief Seattle, 1855

vision board

write your favourite animal quote
stick photo of your favourite animal here

week three

What exercises have I completed and for what duration?
How have my energy levels and moods been affected today?

What foods and portion sizes have I eaten today?
How have my energy levels and moods been affected today?

---

day one

I am grateful for ....

week three

What exercises have I completed and for what duration?
How have my energy levels and moods been affected today?

What foods and portion sizes have I eaten today?
How have my energy levels and moods been affected today?

---

day two

I am ready to let go of ....

....

....

....

....

....

....

....

....

....

....

....

....

....

....

....

....

....

....

....

....

week three

What exercises have I completed and for what duration?
How have my energy levels and moods been affected today?

What foods and portion sizes have I eaten today?
How have my energy levels and moods been affected today?

---

day three

I love my body because ....

yoga

Yoga is more than just a trendy low impact exercise but a holistic approach to health by encompassing the mind, body and spirit. By purifying the body you purify the mind and visa versa.

The ancient practice of Hatha yoga is designed to balance your energy channels so you can find freedom in your body, creating the space to find peace in your mind. Yoga is therefore considered therapeutic. It helps you become more aware of your body's posture, alignment and patterns of movement. It makes the body more flexible and helps you relax even in the midst of a stress stricken environment.

This ancient art has been practiced for over 5000 years and also incorporates breathing practices called pranayama that expand the breath whilst slowing it down. Meditation is a common practice for many yogis seeking to soften the mind, along with conscious awareness and mindfulness in ones daily actions.

This is why people want to start yoga - to feel fit, flexible and more physically energetic whilst being happier and more peaceful emotionally. Other health benefits include reduced blood pressure, anxiety and stress, so why don't you roll out a yoga mat and start stretching yourself to your full potential.

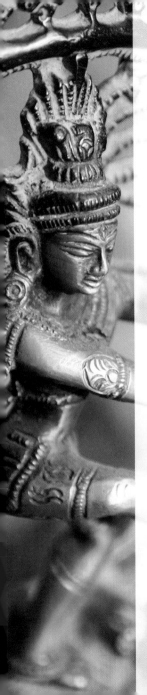

tomato basil spaghetti

Preparation and cooking time: 20 minutes

ingredients

¼ cup (60ml) olive oil
½ onion
teaspoon of garlic
1 cup (250ml) fresh basil, chopped
2 teaspoons (10ml) dried oregano
6 cups (1.5L) tomato puree
1 teaspoon (5ml) salt
¼ teaspoon (1ml) black pepper
1 teaspoon (5ml) raw or brown sugar
2 tablespoons (40ml) tomato paste
4 zucchini

directions

Finely cut onion and cook on medium heat in oil till golden, add garlic and dried oregano. Cook for 2 minutes allow flavours to arise.

Add tomato puree, salt, black pepper, sugar and tomato paste. Cook on medium heat for 10 minutes allowing tomatoes to gently cook.

Add fresh basil and mix well for 5 mins.

Peel the zucchini and make spaghetti on a spiral vegetable slice. Serve with tomato basil sauce.

week three

What exercises have I completed and for what duration?
How have my energy levels and moods been affected today?

_____

_____

_____

_____

_____

_____

_____

_____

What foods and portion sizes have I eaten today?
How have my energy levels and moods been affected today?

_____

_____

_____

_____

_____

_____

day four

I am fearful of _____

_____

_____

_____

_____

_____

_____

_____

_____

_____

_____

_____

_____

_____

_____

_____

_____

_____

_____

_____

_____

week three

What exercises have I completed and for what duration?
How have my energy levels and moods been affected today?

What foods and portion sizes have I eaten today?
How have my energy levels and moods been affected today?

---

day five

My dreams and plans are

day five

My dreams and plans are

week three

What exercises have I completed and for what duration?
How have my energy levels and moods been affected today?

What foods and portion sizes have I eaten today?
How have my energy levels and moods been affected today?

Today I made someone happy because

week three

What exercises have I completed and for what duration?
How have my energy levels and moods been affected today?

What foods and portion sizes have I eaten today?
How have my energy levels and moods been affected today?

I will change the world by

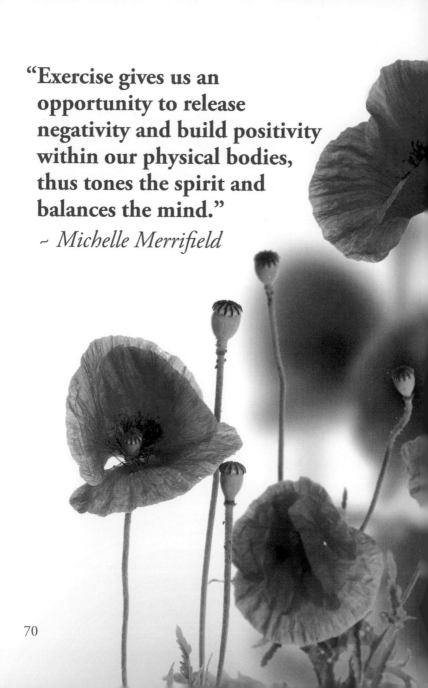

"Exercise gives us an opportunity to release negativity and build positivity within our physical bodies, thus tones the spirit and balances the mind."

~ *Michelle Merrifield*

vision board

write your favourite exercise quote
stick a photo of someone doing your favourite exercise here

week four

What exercises have I completed and for what duration?
How have my energy levels and moods been affected today?

_____

_____

_____

_____

_____

_____

_____

_____

_____

What foods and portion sizes have I eaten today?
How have my energy levels and moods been affected today?

_____

_____

_____

_____

_____

_____

_____

day one

I am grateful for

week four

What exercises have I completed and for what duration?
How have my energy levels and moods been affected today?

What foods and portion sizes have I eaten today?
How have my energy levels and moods been affected today?

----

day two

I am ready to let go of

week four

What exercises have I completed and for what duration?
How have my energy levels and moods been affected today?

_____

_____

_____

_____

_____

_____

_____

_____

What foods and portion sizes have I eaten today?
How have my energy levels and moods been affected today?

_____

_____

_____

_____

_____

_____

day three

I love my body because _____

_____

_____

_____

_____

_____

_____

_____

_____

_____

_____

_____

_____

_____

_____

_____

_____

_____

_____

_____

_____

_____

running

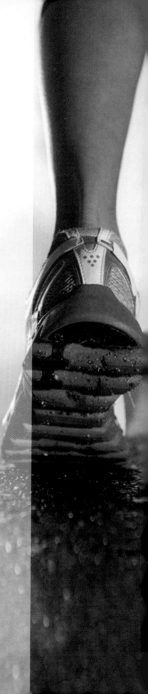

Human beings started walking and running some 4-6 million years ago when we evolved and rose from all fours. Ten thousand years ago hunter-gatherers ran 24-120 kilometers a day on the hunt, but it was Pheidippides (490 BC), an ancient "day-runner," who put running on the map. He is said to have run 240 kilometers to carry the news of the Persian landing at Marathon to Sparta in order to enlist help for the battle. It was in his honor the marathon (42 kilometers) was born, with its first appearance being in the modern Olympic Games of 1896 in Athens.

The Merriam-Webster dictionary definition of running is: 'to go steadily by springing steps so that both feet leave the ground for an instant in each step.' Often people dislike running due to lack of confidence in their speed or abilities, however running has nothing to do with how quick you are, as the key is to have both feet in the air at once. Start by taking it slow and steady and gradually as your fitness improves, you will begin to run faster and further.

Beware running can be addictive, the runners high is a well coined term that comes from the feeling of flying across the earth and clearing your mind promoting a sense of freedom and empowerment within.

italian eggplant, tomato & chickpea

Preparation and cooking time: 30 minutes

ingredients
2 medium eggplants, washed
1 cup oil (not olive oil)
¼ cup olive oil
½ onion
1 teaspoon garlic
3 ripe tomatoes, peeled, seeded and chopped
1 tablespoon tomato paste
½ cup water
1 teaspoon salt
½ teaspoon freshly ground pepper
2 cups chickpeas

directions
Cut the eggplants into strips.

Heat the oil in fry pan on moderate to high heat. When the oil is hot, add enough eggplant strips to fill frying pan. Shallow-fry the eggplant until soft. Remove the eggplant from pan with a spoon and drain.

Heat olive oil in separate frying pan. When oil is hot, cook onion and garlic till golden, add tomatoes, tomato paste and water. Cook uncovered for 10 minutes or until sauce is thick.

Add salt and pepper, mix well, and add eggplant and chickpeas. Serve either hot or cold.

week four

What exercises have I completed and for what duration?
How have my energy levels and moods been affected today?

What foods and portion sizes have I eaten today?
How have my energy levels and moods been affected today?

----

day four

I am fearful of _____

_____

_____

_____

_____

_____

_____

_____

_____

_____

_____

_____

_____

_____

_____

_____

_____

_____

_____

_____

week four

What exercises have I completed and for what duration?
How have my energy levels and moods been affected today?

_____

_____

_____

_____

_____

_____

_____

_____

What foods and portion sizes have I eaten today?
How have my energy levels and moods been affected today?

_____

_____

_____

_____

_____

_____

day five

My dreams and plans are

week four

What exercises have I completed and for what duration?
How have my energy levels and moods been affected today?

What foods and portion sizes have I eaten today?
How have my energy levels and moods been affected today?

----

day six

Today I made someone happy because

week four

What exercises have I completed and for what duration?
How have my energy levels and moods been affected today?

_____

_____

_____

_____

_____

_____

_____

_____

What foods and portion sizes have I eaten today?
How have my energy levels and moods been affected today?

_____

_____

_____

_____

_____

_____

day seven

I will change the world by _____

_____

_____

_____

_____

_____

_____

_____

_____

_____

_____

_____

_____

_____

_____

_____

_____

_____

_____

_____

_____

_____

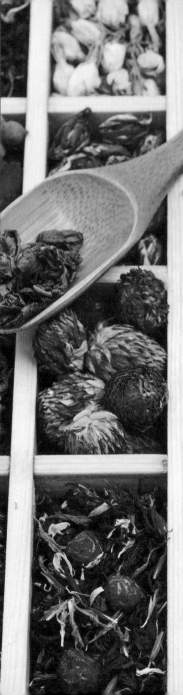

Let food be
thy medicine
and medicine
be thy food.

~ *Hippocrates*

vision board

write your favourite quote about food
stick a photo of your favourite food here

week five

What exercises have I completed and for what duration?
How have my energy levels and moods been affected today?

What foods and portion sizes have I eaten today?
How have my energy levels and moods been affected today?

----

day one

I am grateful for

week five

What exercises have I completed and for what duration?
How have my energy levels and moods been affected today?

_____
_____
_____
_____
_____
_____
_____
_____
_____

What foods and portion sizes have I eaten today?
How have my energy levels and moods been affected today?

_____
_____
_____
_____
_____
_____
_____

day two

I am ready to let go of

week five

What exercises have I completed and for what duration?
How have my energy levels and moods been affected today?

_____

_____

_____

_____

_____

_____

_____

_____

_____

What foods and portion sizes have I eaten today?
How have my energy levels and moods been affected today?

_____

_____

_____

_____

_____

_____

day three

I love my body because

cleaning

Cleanliness is next to godliness but it's also next to gorgeousness. Not only does cleaning your house make you feel good about having a clutter free home, cleaning anything in general burns calories. You can burn an average of 205 calories an hour during a cleaning frenzy—even more if you're really moving. Busting out that vacuum cleaner can also help you drop those extra pounds or make that stress melt away. With all these health benefits, why wouldn't you want to clean every week (or even every day)? Research the top calorie-burning chores to make sure you maximize your "workout" potential.

Cleaning can also eliminate your daily sneeze attacks. By purging your home of those dust mites, you can improve or avoid allergies and hay fever entirely. Frequently vacuuming, washing your sheets and curtains, cleaning out your sink & refrigerator and thoroughly dusting your furniture, are among the best ways to control your allergies. Your annual spring clean is the perfect time to really reach those nooks and crannies that you rarely get to otherwise. Why not spring clean every season? Taking time now will save you headaches (and itchy, red eyes) later.

In 2008, an article published in the British Journal of Sports Medicine stated that twenty minutes of housework cuts anxiety and stress by as much as 20 percent. After all, if you know where to find your car keys for instance, you can completely bypass that frantic and stressful search right before work.

I dare you to start with just one room at a time for just 10 minutes and see how good it makes you feel inside and out. Only 10 minutes of cleaning before you leave for work and 10 minutes before you go to bed can change your life and your body.

cauliflower soup

Preparation and Ccooking time:
30 minutes

ingredients
Nuttelex
half an onion
1 large cauliflower
½ teaspoon of curry powder
1 litre of vegetable stock
2 bay leaves
Salt & pepper to taste
Fresh coriander
(use as much as you like)

directions
Melt Nuttelex, add onion and
curry powder and cook for
10 minutes on low heat.

Add vegetable stock and small
cauliflower pieces, drop 2 bay leaves
into stock and cook for 15 minutes
on low heat with the lid on.

Add salt, pepper and coriander as
desired.

Simmer for 5 minutes then blend.

97

week five

What exercises have I completed and for what duration?
How have my energy levels and moods been affected today?

What foods and portion sizes have I eaten today?
How have my energy levels and moods been affected today?

----

day four

I am fearful of _____

week five

What exercises have I completed and for what duration?
How have my energy levels and moods been affected today?

What foods and portion sizes have I eaten today?
How have my energy levels and moods been affected today?

---

day five

My dreams and plans are

week five

What exercises have I completed and for what duration?
How have my energy levels and moods been affected today?

What foods and portion sizes have I eaten today?
How have my energy levels and moods been affected today?

----

day six

Today I made someone happy because

week five

What exercises have I completed and for what duration?
How have my energy levels and moods been affected today?

_____

_____

_____

_____

_____

_____

_____

_____

What foods and portion sizes have I eaten today?
How have my energy levels and moods been affected today?

_____

_____

_____

_____

_____

_____

day seven

I will change the world by _____

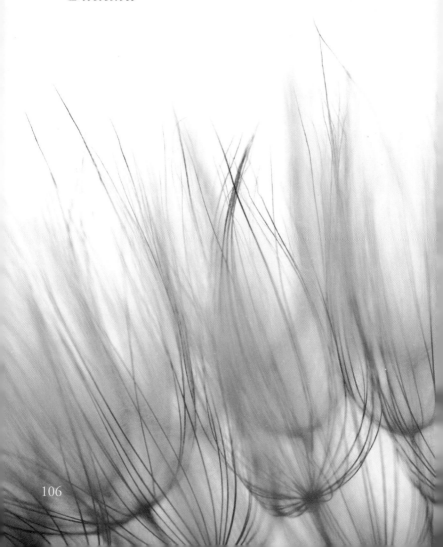

"As you think so you are,
   as you imagine so you become."

- *Buddha*

vision board

write your favourite quote from someone who inspires you here
stick a photo of someone who inspires you

week six

What exercises have I completed and for what duration?
How have my energy levels and moods been affected today?

_____

_____

_____

_____

_____

_____

_____

_____

_____

What foods and portion sizes have I eaten today?
How have my energy levels and moods been affected today?

_____

_____

_____

_____

_____

_____

_____

day one

I am grateful for

week six

What exercises have I completed and for what duration?
How have my energy levels and moods been affected today?

What foods and portion sizes have I eaten today?
How have my energy levels and moods been affected today?

----

day two

I am ready to let go of

week six

What exercises have I completed and for what duration?
How have my energy levels and moods been affected today?

What foods and portion sizes have I eaten today?
How have my energy levels and moods been affected today?

----

day three

I love my body because _____

taking the stairs

Given all our modern conveniences including cars, elevators, escalators and computers, it is easy to go through a whole day without getting much physical activity.

Activities that you can fit into your daily routine – like choosing the stairs instead of the elevator – is increasingly being urged by public health experts who point to mounting evidence that small amounts of exercise accumulated throughout the day can provide significant health benefits. Stair climbing is a 'green' activity; the only energy source used is what is stored in our bodies... good for you and the environment!

Taking the stairs is an excellent way to prevent the health problems that develop through inactivity such as obesity, high blood pressure, heart disease and stroke. Taking the stairs is a great way to get into shape, improve cardiovascular function and strengthen and tone the leg muscles. Taking the stairs requires no special skills, equipment or clothing yet it burns twice as many calories as walking.

So the next time you find yourself standing at the proverbial fork in the road having to choose between an elevator and a flight of stairs, take the stairs and your body will thank you for it. So step right up!

vegan pizza & cashew cheese

Preparation and cooking time: 40 minutes

spelt pizza crust
(wheat free ingredients)
- 2 cups of light spelt flour
- 1 ½ half teaspoons quick-rising yeast
- 1 teaspoon baking powder
- 1 ¼ tablespoons olive oil
- 1 teaspoon honey
- ⅔ cup of warm water
- ¾ teaspoon of salt

directions

Stir first 3 ingredients together.

Add remaining ingredients and stir well.

Kneed until smooth.

Stretch to fit greased 10 or 12 inch pizza pan.

Place in oven 180°C till golden.

Remove and add toppings of choice. We recommend:
- Marinated semi dried tomatoes
- Roasted eggplant
- Roasted artichoke
- Sliced kalamata olives
- Cashew cheese

Spinach leaves on last to garnish.

cashew cheese ingredients
- 1 ½ cups raw not roasted/unsalted cashews
- ¼ of filtered water
- 2 tablespoons freshly squeezed lemon juice
- 1 teaspoon white wine vinegar
- 2 tablespoons nutritional yeast
- 2 gloves of garlic
- ½ teaspoon Himalayan sea salt
- Freshly ground pepper

directions

Soak cashews 2-3 hours.

Add all ingredients together.

Mix using food processor.

Leave it in the fridge over night.

Spread out over the pizza then put in the oven 180°C.

115

week six

What exercises have I completed and for what duration?
How have my energy levels and moods been affected today?

What foods and portion sizes have I eaten today?
How have my energy levels and moods been affected today?

---

day four

I am fearful of

week six

What exercises have I completed and for what duration?
How have my energy levels and moods been affected today?

What foods and portion sizes have I eaten today?
How have my energy levels and moods been affected today?

----

day five

My dreams and plans are

week six

What exercises have I completed and for what duration?
How have my energy levels and moods been affected today?

_____

_____

_____

_____

_____

_____

_____

_____

What foods and portion sizes have I eaten today?
How have my energy levels and moods been affected today?

_____

_____

_____

_____

_____

_____

day six

Today I made someone happy because

week six

What exercises have I completed and for what duration?
How have my energy levels and moods been affected today?

_____

_____

_____

_____

_____

_____

_____

_____

What foods and portion sizes have I eaten today?
How have my energy levels and moods been affected today?

_____

_____

_____

_____

_____

_____

day seven

I will change the world by ....

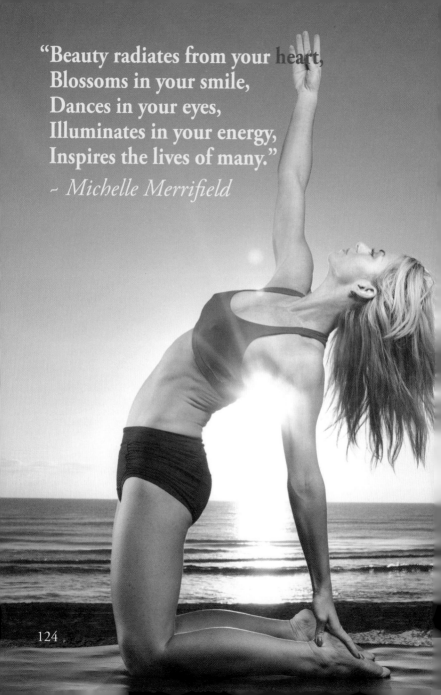

"Beauty radiates from your heart,
Blossoms in your smile,
Dances in your eyes,
Illuminates in your energy,
Inspires the lives of many."

~ Michelle Merrifield

124

vision board

write your favourite body quote
stick a photo of your inspirational body here

week seven

What exercises have I completed and for what duration?
How have my energy levels and moods been affected today?

What foods and portion sizes have I eaten today?
How have my energy levels and moods been affected today?

---

day one

I am grateful for

week seven

What exercises have I completed and for what duration?
How have my energy levels and moods been affected today?

What foods and portion sizes have I eaten today?
How have my energy levels and moods been affected today?

----

day two

I am ready to let go of

week seven

What exercises have I completed and for what duration?
How have my energy levels and moods been affected today?

What foods and portion sizes have I eaten today?
How have my energy levels and moods been affected today?

---

day three

I love my body because ....

pilates

'Pilates' originates from the founder's surname: Joseph Pilates. His style of training is about 100 years old comprising of a series of over 500 mat or and equipment based exercises inspired by calisthenics, yoga and ballet. Pilates improves flexibility, strength, balance, and body awareness. Pilates was originally designed to help injured soldiers during the war and was later introduced to America during the 1920's as a way to assist injured athletes and dancers to safely return to exercise and maintain their fitness levels.

Since then, Pilates has been adapted to suit people in the general community. Pilates can be an aerobic or anaerobic form of exercise. It requires concentration as the body moves through precise ranges of motion with control and focus. There are two types of Pilates commonly practiced today;

1. Pilates for Rehabilitation instructed by Physiotherapists performing controlled slow equipment based exercises.
2. Pilates for Fitness often instructed by dancers and physical trainers performing more dynamic faster floor based and small apparatus exercises.

With two very popular styles of Pilates available, practice is easily accessible to the wider community ensuring that everyone can reap the health benefits from this method. Some of the benefits that make Pilates so popular are the greater awareness of postural alignment and strengthening practices, along with improved coordination and balance.

Pilates is famous for its coined term the powerhouse focusing its method based on the buttocks, hips, lower back and abdominals for stability and safety of movement. So if you want a wash board tummy and tight toned thighs, Pilates is the practice for you.

132

acai bowls

Preparation time: 10 minutes

ingredients
Acai puree or sachets
(available from Health food
store freezer sections)
Pre-freeze one whole ripe banana
½ can coconut water

directions
Scoop desired amount of acai puree
into blender with banana and blend.

To assist with the blending, slowly
add coconut water. If at any point it
gets a little thick, add coconut water
as desired to smooth over the texture.

Serve in an ice-cream bowl.

week seven

What exercises have I completed and for what duration?
How have my energy levels and moods been affected today?

_____

_____

_____

_____

_____

_____

_____

_____

What foods and portion sizes have I eaten today?
How have my energy levels and moods been affected today?

_____

_____

_____

_____

_____

_____

day four

I am fearful of

week seven

What exercises have I completed and for what duration?
How have my energy levels and moods been affected today?

What foods and portion sizes have I eaten today?
How have my energy levels and moods been affected today?

----

day five

My dreams and plans are

week seven

What exercises have I completed and for what duration?
How have my energy levels and moods been affected today?

What foods and portion sizes have I eaten today?
How have my energy levels and moods been affected today?

----

day six

Today I made someone happy because _____

_____

_____

_____

_____

_____

_____

_____

_____

_____

_____

_____

_____

_____

_____

_____

_____

_____

_____

_____

week seven

What exercises have I completed and for what duration?
How have my energy levels and moods been affected today?

What foods and portion sizes have I eaten today?
How have my energy levels and moods been affected today?

----

day seven

I will change the world by _____

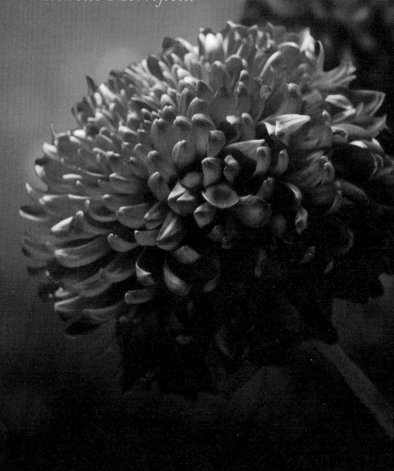

"Stay in-tune, in-touch and in-sync with universal vibration."

– *Michelle Merrifield*

vision board

write your favourite musical lyric
stick a photo of your favourite musician here

week eight

What exercises have I completed and for what duration?
How have my energy levels and moods been affected today?

_____

_____

_____

_____

_____

_____

_____

_____

What foods and portion sizes have I eaten today?
How have my energy levels and moods been affected today?

_____

_____

_____

_____

_____

_____

day one

I am grateful for _____

_____

_____

_____

_____

_____

_____

_____

_____

_____

_____

_____

_____

_____

_____

_____

_____

_____

week eight

What exercises have I completed and for what duration?
How have my energy levels and moods been affected today?

_____

_____

_____

_____

_____

_____

_____

_____

What foods and portion sizes have I eaten today?
How have my energy levels and moods been affected today?

_____

_____

_____

_____

_____

_____

day two

I am ready to let go of _____

_____

_____

_____

_____

_____

_____

_____

_____

_____

_____

_____

_____

_____

_____

_____

_____

_____

_____

_____

_____

week eight

What exercises have I completed and for what duration?
How have my energy levels and moods been affected today?

What foods and portion sizes have I eaten today?
How have my energy levels and moods been affected today?

day three

I love my body because _____

singing

Music is the "universal language" stirring our deepest emotions, improving our health and energy levels, widening our communities and enriching our imaginations. It can carry us through even the most stress-filled life commitments demonstrating multiple benefits from singing: physically, emotionally and socially.

Singing not only exercises our lungs, it tones our intercostal muscles and diaphragms promoting superior posture that triggers our sinuses and respiratory tubes to open up more. Studies have shown that with careful training it can help decrease the problem of snoring and is proven to help us sleep better at night.

Singing has the power to shift our state of mind and mood in an instant. As soon as you hear your favourite song your emotional state is instantly elevated, it's that powerful. Singing has the ability to motivate and energise you so you feel as though you could do anything. It touches your spirit and increases feelings of wellbeing and positivity.

Singing is an excellent outlet for expressive creativity and communication. It can reduce stress and heal us emotionally by increasing our self-esteem and confidence. It increases our ability to understand and empathise with other cultures and people, promoting bonding and connecting with others through song.

So start singing in the shower or turn up your radio and sing along to your favorite song or why not get creative and write your own lyrics and start singing your own story today. Singing will keep your body and soul in tune.

savory chickpeas

Preparation and cooking time: 15 minutes

ingredients
1¼ cups chickpeas
3 tablespoons (60ml) olive oil
½ teaspoon (2ml) mustard seeds
1½ teaspoons (7ml) cumin seeds
1½ teaspoons (7ml) minced fresh ginger
1½ teaspoons (7ml) fresh green chillies, seeded and chopped
10 fresh curry leaves
1¾ cups (435ml) ripe, finely-chopped tomatoes, about 5 medium tomatoes
1 teaspoon (7ml) turmeric
¼ cup (60ml) chopped fresh coriander leaves
1½ teaspoon (7ml) chat masala
½ teaspoon (2ml) garam masala
1¼ teaspoon (6ml) salt
1 teaspoon (20ml) nuttlex

directions
In a 2L saucepan, prepare the tomato glaze as follows: warm the oil over moderate heat. When fairly hot but not smoking, drop in the mustard seeds. When they crackle and then greyish, add the cumin. As the cumin darkens a few shades, drop in the ginger, chillies and curry leaves. Stir-fry the spices for 1 or 2 mins or until the spices are fragrant.

Add the chopped tomatoes, turmeric, half the coriander, chat masala and the garam masala. Cook, stirring occasionally for 5-7mins, or oil oozes out and the tomatoes are broken down and saucy.

Drain the chickpeas, reserving the cooking water. Stir the chickpeas into the sauce reduce the heat to low and cook for another 10 mins more, adding a little chickpeas moist.

Remove the savoury glazed chickpeas from the heat, add the remaining nuttlex, salt and the rest of the herbs.

Serve hot with wedges of lemon or lime and pappadams.

week eight

What exercises have I completed and for what duration?
How have my energy levels and moods been affected today?

_____

_____

_____

_____

_____

_____

_____

_____

_____

_____

What foods and portion sizes have I eaten today?
How have my energy levels and moods been affected today?

_____

_____

_____

_____

_____

_____

I am fearful of ....

----

week eight

What exercises have I completed and for what duration?
How have my energy levels and moods been affected today?

What foods and portion sizes have I eaten today?
How have my energy levels and moods been affected today?

----

day five

My dreams and plans are

week eight

What exercises have I completed and for what duration?
How have my energy levels and moods been affected today?

What foods and portion sizes have I eaten today?
How have my energy levels and moods been affected today?

-----

day six

Today I made someone happy because _____

week eight

What exercises have I completed and for what duration?
How have my energy levels and moods been affected today?

_____

_____

_____

_____

_____

_____

_____

_____

What foods and portion sizes have I eaten today?
How have my energy levels and moods been affected today?

_____

_____

_____

_____

_____

_____

day seven

I will change the world by _____

_____

_____

_____

_____

_____

_____

_____

_____

_____

_____

_____

_____

_____

_____

_____

_____

_____

_____

_____

_____

"The real voyage of discovery consists
not in seeking new landscapes,
but in having new eyes."

~ *Marcel Proust*

vision board

write your favourite travel quote
stick a photo of your dream holiday here

week nine

What exercises have I completed and for what duration?
How have my energy levels and moods been affected today?

What foods and portion sizes have I eaten today?
How have my energy levels and moods been affected today?

----

day one

I am grateful for

week nine

What exercises have I completed and for what duration?
How have my energy levels and moods been affected today?

_____

_____

_____

_____

_____

_____

_____

_____

What foods and portion sizes have I eaten today?
How have my energy levels and moods been affected today?

_____

_____

_____

_____

_____

_____

day two

I am ready to let go of _____

_____

_____

_____

_____

_____

_____

_____

_____

_____

_____

_____

_____

_____

_____

_____

_____

_____

_____

_____

week nine

What exercises have I completed and for what duration?
How have my energy levels and moods been affected today?

What foods and portion sizes have I eaten today?
How have my energy levels and moods been affected today?

----

day three

I love my body because

bike riding

Most of us know how to ride a bike and once you have learned you don't forget. Bike riding is a great way to exercise whilst also enjoying the environment around you. Cycling is mainly an aerobic activity, meaning your heart, blood vessels and lungs all get a workout. It can be viewed as a highly competitive sport however you may just want to be a casual cruiser cycling the great outdoors to be one with nature and to feel the breath of the earth.

Cycling can be done as an environmentally friendly form of transport or for fun shared with family and friends. Riding a bike is enjoyed by people of all ages, all over the world. There are many amazing cycling holidays you can experience around the world which can be a great opportunity to meet new people and discover new places.

Cycling is a great way to 'escape' from worries and everyday stresses of life as jumping on your bike with the wind in your hair rejuvenates your soul and clears your mind. Cycling is both low impact and low cost that can be done at anytime, anywhere, all year round. All it takes is a roadworthy bike, a helmet and some pedal power.

So dust off your bike and enjoy the ride of your life.

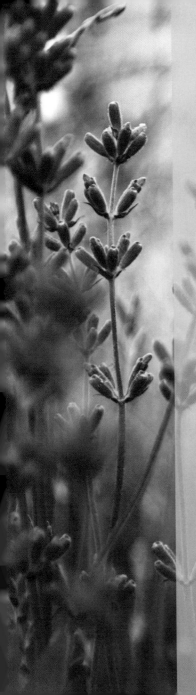

banana
smoothie

Preparation time: 5 minutes

ingredients
½L oat milk
2 tbsp of chia seeds
2 tbsp of LSA
(linseed, sunflower
seed & almond meal)
2 bananas
6 medjool dates
Handful of ice to your pleasing

directions
Add all ingredients to a blender
and blend till smooth.

Drink immediately for optimal
nutrition.

week nine

What exercises have I completed and for what duration?
How have my energy levels and moods been affected today?

_____

_____

_____

_____

_____

_____

_____

_____

What foods and portion sizes have I eaten today?
How have my energy levels and moods been affected today?

_____

_____

_____

_____

_____

day four

I am fearful of

week nine

What exercises have I completed and for what duration?
How have my energy levels and moods been affected today?

What foods and portion sizes have I eaten today?
How have my energy levels and moods been affected today?

----

day five

My dreams and plans are

week nine

What exercises have I completed and for what duration?
How have my energy levels and moods been affected today?

What foods and portion sizes have I eaten today?
How have my energy levels and moods been affected today?

day six

Today I made someone happy because

week nine

What exercises have I completed and for what duration?
How have my energy levels and moods been affected today?

What foods and portion sizes have I eaten today?
How have my energy levels and moods been affected today?

---

day seven

I will change the world by

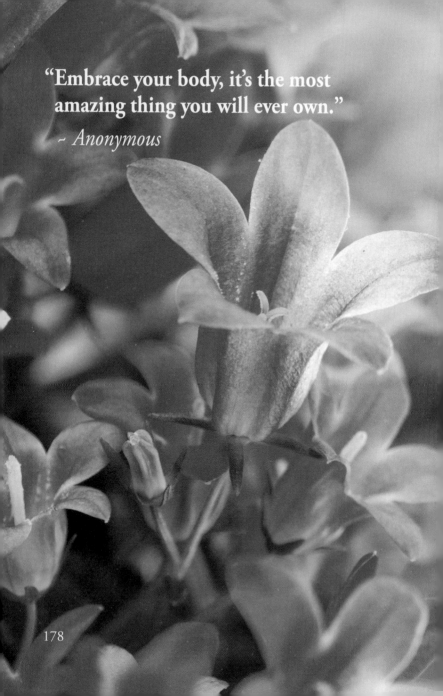

"Embrace your body, it's the most amazing thing you will ever own."

- *Anonymous*

178

vision board

write what you love about your body
stick a photo of you happy & healthy here

week ten

What exercises have I completed and for what duration?
How have my energy levels and moods been affected today?

What foods and portion sizes have I eaten today?
How have my energy levels and moods been affected today?

----

day one

I am grateful for

week ten

What exercises have I completed and for what duration?
How have my energy levels and moods been affected today?

What foods and portion sizes have I eaten today?
How have my energy levels and moods been affected today?

----

day two

I am ready to let go of

week ten

What exercises have I completed and for what duration?
How have my energy levels and moods been affected today?

_____

_____

_____

_____

_____

_____

_____

_____

What foods and portion sizes have I eaten today?
How have my energy levels and moods been affected today?

_____

_____

_____

_____

_____

_____

day three

I love my body because

dancing

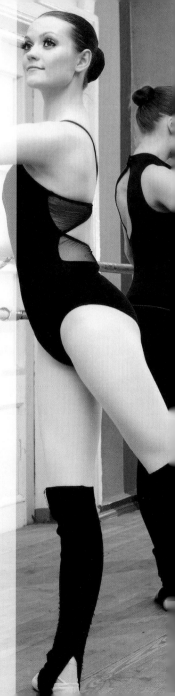

Dancers are often acknowledged for their agile ageless bodies. They have a sense of poise and grace as they float into a room with toned bodies and perfect posture. They move smoothly with an incredible inner strength.

Two of the greatest benefits of dancing is flexibility and balance; a dancer strives to achieve full range of movement in all major muscle groups whilst staying centred and balanced. This serves to increase the overall quality of modern day life, as they age and continue to move, twist and turn as life demands.

Dancing is an excellent way to increase your fitness as it increases your heart rate, stamina and is a calorie blaster. Simply dancing in your lounge room is a fun safe way to move the body in a large dynamic way, activating a diverse range of muscles promoting strong healthy bones.

Dancing is like singing; it is an art and a form of self-expression for many keen enthusiasts. It is universal and has no cultural barriers. People from all parts of the world with different ideologies, meet on the dance floor and it's a great way to make new friends and build social skills giving you a sense of well being.

186

super salad

Preparation and cooking Time: 15 minutes

ingredients
- ½ cos lettuce
- 1 tomato
- 1 avocado
- 1 cup mung-bean sprouts
- ½ cup of diced kalamata olives
- 1 small broccoli (raw, finely chopped)
- ½ carrot (grated)
- ½ beetroot (grated)
- ¾ cup walnuts (dry pan roasted in honey)
- Asian salad dressing – as desired

directions
Prepare grated vegetables, sprouts, dice broccoli, olives & tomato as desired.

Roughly tear cos lettuce and combine with vegetables in a large mixing bowl.

Season with dressing to your taste.

Lastly, decorate with your candied walnuts.

candied walnuts ingredients
- ½ cup honey
- ½ teaspoon sea salt (optional)
- 1 cup unbroken walnut halves
- ¼ teaspoon cayenne pepper (optional)

directions
Combine honey, salt and cayenne in a small pot over medium heat.

Stir once then cook 3 minutes till candying begins.

Add walnuts, stir to coat.

Simmer 5–7 minutes or until syrup is lightly browned.

Place walnuts on a pan to bake in moderate oven 180 C for about 8 minutes or until nuts have darkened slightly (this prevents them from sogging).

Once removed from the over the nuts will crisp as they cool.

week ten

What exercises have I completed and for what duration?
How have my energy levels and moods been affected today?

_____

_____

_____

_____

_____

_____

_____

_____

What foods and portion sizes have I eaten today?
How have my energy levels and moods been affected today?

_____

_____

_____

_____

_____

_____

day four

I am fearful of

week ten

What exercises have I completed and for what duration?
How have my energy levels and moods been affected today?

What foods and portion sizes have I eaten today?
How have my energy levels and moods been affected today?

----

day five

My dreams and plans are

week ten

What exercises have I completed and for what duration?
How have my energy levels and moods been affected today?

What foods and portion sizes have I eaten today?
How have my energy levels and moods been affected today?

----

day six

Today I made someone happy because _____

week ten

What exercises have I completed and for what duration?
How have my energy levels and moods been affected today?

What foods and portion sizes have I eaten today?
How have my energy levels and moods been affected today?

194

day seven

I will change the world by _____

_____

_____

_____

_____

_____

_____

_____

_____

_____

_____

_____

_____

_____

_____

_____

_____

_____

_____

_____

_____

_____

_____

"We return thanks to our mother,
the earth, which sustains us.
We return thanks to the rivers
and streams, which supply us
with water.
We return thanks to all herbs,
which furnish medicines for
the cure of our diseases.
We return thanks to the moon
and stars, which have given to us
their light when the sun was gone.
We return thanks to the sun, that
has looked upon the earth with
a beneficent eye.
Lastly, we return thanks to the
Great Spirit, in Whom is
embodied all goodness, and
Who directs all things for the
good of Her children."

~ Iroquois

vision board

write your favourite place in nature
stick a photo of nature that inspires you

week eleven

What exercises have I completed and for what duration?
How have my energy levels and moods been affected today?

_____

_____

_____

_____

_____

_____

_____

_____

What foods and portion sizes have I eaten today?
How have my energy levels and moods been affected today?

_____

_____

_____

_____

_____

_____

day one

I am grateful for _____

_____

_____

_____

_____

_____

_____

_____

_____

_____

_____

_____

_____

_____

_____

_____

_____

_____

_____

_____

_____

week eleven

What exercises have I completed and for what duration?
How have my energy levels and moods been affected today?

What foods and portion sizes have I eaten today?
How have my energy levels and moods been affected today?

---

day two

I am ready to let go of _____

_____

_____

_____

_____

_____

_____

_____

_____

_____

_____

_____

_____

_____

_____

_____

_____

_____

_____

week eleven

What exercises have I completed and for what duration?
How have my energy levels and moods been affected today?

What foods and portion sizes have I eaten today?
How have my energy levels and moods been affected today?

---

day three

I love my body because _____

_____

_____

_____

_____

_____

_____

_____

_____

_____

_____

_____

_____

_____

_____

_____

_____

_____

_____

_____

_____

hiking

Walking on a treadmill can get tedious, so hiking in the great outdoors provides a welcomed break from the fluorescent lights and mirrors of a gymnasium. There's something therapeutic about being outdoors and in the presence of nature. Whether you hike alone or with a friend, you'll feel your worries melt away as you absorb the sunshine and breathe in the fresh air. If it's a sunny day, you'll also get a healthy dose of vitamin D, also known as the sunshine vitamin.

The great thing about hiking is you can choose a different path each day to keep your workout fresh and interesting. With the ever changing scenery and the sweet smell of fresh air to inspire and motivate you, you'll never get bored of this type of exercise. In fact they found that taking a hike in the countryside reduces depression, whereas walking in a shopping centre increases depression.

Even though hiking can be a tough workout, depending upon the terrain you choose, there's minimal stress on the joints since you're never lifting more than one foot off the ground at a time. You get an excellent toning workout for the lower body when you hike, particularly if you choose trails with hills and elevations.

If you live in a city, why not utilise your weekends by jumping in a car and venturing into the wild so you may experience nature up close and personal whilst getting a great workout.

popeye power

Preparation and cooking time: 15 minutes

ingredients
1kg fresh spinach
1 tablespoon (20ml) olive oil
½ cup (85ml) pine nuts
½ cup (125ml) seeded raisins
¾ teaspoon (3ml) salt
Freshly-grounded black pepper

directions
Cut off the roots and base of the stems of spinach and discard them.

Place the leaves in a sink or large bowl filled with cool water.

Remove the leaves to a colander and rinse under cold running water.

Pat the leaves dry or shake them well.

Place the spinach in a covered 5-litre saucepan and cook over low heat for 5 minutes or until the spinach leaves are softened.

Heat the oil in a pan or wok over moderate heat. When the oil is fairly hot, drop in the pine nuts and stir them for 1 or 2 minutes, or until lightly golden.

Add the raisins and stir until they are plump and puffed. Add the spinach and salt, and toss quickly over high heat.

Sprinkle with the ground black pepper and serve immediately.

week eleven

What exercises have I completed and for what duration?
How have my energy levels and moods been affected today?

What foods and portion sizes have I eaten today?
How have my energy levels and moods been affected today?

---

day four

I am fearful of

week eleven

What exercises have I completed and for what duration?
How have my energy levels and moods been affected today?

_____

_____

_____

_____

_____

_____

_____

_____

What foods and portion sizes have I eaten today?
How have my energy levels and moods been affected today?

_____

_____

_____

_____

_____

_____

day five

My dreams and plans are

week eleven

What exercises have I completed and for what duration?
How have my energy levels and moods been affected today?

_____

_____

_____

_____

_____

_____

_____

_____

What foods and portion sizes have I eaten today?
How have my energy levels and moods been affected today?

_____

_____

_____

_____

_____

_____

day six

Today I made someone happy because

week eleven

What exercises have I completed and for what duration?
How have my energy levels and moods been affected today?

What foods and portion sizes have I eaten today?
How have my energy levels and moods been affected today?

----

day seven

I will change the world by _____

_____

_____

_____

_____

_____

_____

_____

_____

_____

_____

_____

_____

_____

_____

_____

_____

_____

_____

_____

_____

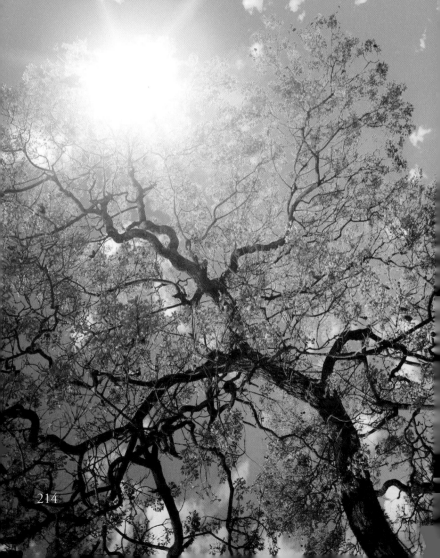

"Dream your dreams with open eyes
and make them come true."

- *T E Lawrence*

vision board

write your dreams
stick a photo of your dreams here

week twelve

What exercises have I completed and for what duration?
How have my energy levels and moods been affected today?

_____

_____

_____

_____

_____

_____

_____

_____

_____

What foods and portion sizes have I eaten today?
How have my energy levels and moods been affected today?

_____

_____

_____

_____

_____

_____

_____

day one

I am grateful for _____

week twelve

What exercises have I completed and for what duration?
How have my energy levels and moods been affected today?

_____
_____
_____
_____
_____
_____
_____
_____

What foods and portion sizes have I eaten today?
How have my energy levels and moods been affected today?

_____
_____
_____
_____
_____
_____

day two

I am ready to let go of ⸻

week twelve

What exercises have I completed and for what duration?
How have my energy levels and moods been affected today?

_____

_____

_____

_____

_____

_____

_____

_____

What foods and portion sizes have I eaten today?
How have my energy levels and moods been affected today?

_____

_____

_____

_____

_____

_____

_____

day three

I love my body because

sleeping

Who would have thought sleeping helps you lose weight? Researchers have found that people who sleep less than seven hours per night are more likely to be overweight or obese. It is thought that the lack of sleep impacts the balance of hormones in the body that affect appetite. So if you want to control or lose weight make sure you get a good night's sleep.

It is when we are asleep that our bodies have the precious time to heal and repair damage caused by stress, ultra violet rays and other dangerous exposures we may be faced with day to day. Your cells produce more protein while you are sleeping and it's the protein molecules that form the building blocks for cells, which allows them to heal and repair.

Sleeping is where dreams are made. It is where our conscious minds settles and our sub conscious mind manifests. Try and sleep at least 7-8 hours a night to keep the body and mind happy and healthy as sleeping helps fight depression and heart disease.

An afternoon catnap also has many health benefits and is an excellent and effective alternative to caffeine; it can improve your health and make you more productive. A study done in Greek adults showed people who napped had a lower risk for dying from heart disease and had lower levels of stress. Napping improves your memory, cognitive function and mood.

asian salad

Preparation and cooking time: 15 minutes

ingredients
1/2 fancy lettuce broken up
200g pine nuts roasted till golden then add 200g cranberry for
2 minutes on medium heat
Half bunch mint finely cut
Half bunch coriander finely cut
1 punnett cherry tomato cut into quarters
1 small spanish onion finely cut
1 small bag bean sprouts
2 avocado
6 mushrooms finely cut & stir fried till cooked
Balsamic vinegar to taste

directions
Tear or finely slice lettuce, fresh herbs depending on your desired outcome.

Finely dice mushrooms and pan fry in the lightest amount of coconut oil.

Dice avocado and tomatoes a into small pieces.

Thinly dice onion.

Toss in bean sprouts.

Dry roast (meaning oil free) pine nuts on a low heat stovetop pan until golden, then toss in cranberries for a few moments to warm, stir constantly.

Drizzle balsamic vinegar to taste and stir evenly.

week twelve

What exercises have I completed and for what duration?
How have my energy levels and moods been affected today?

_____

_____

_____

_____

_____

_____

_____

_____

_____

What foods and portion sizes have I eaten today?
How have my energy levels and moods been affected today?

_____

_____

_____

_____

_____

_____

_____

day four

I am fearful of _____

_____

_____

_____

_____

_____

_____

_____

_____

_____

_____

_____

_____

_____

_____

_____

_____

_____

_____

_____

week twelve

What exercises have I completed and for what duration?
How have my energy levels and moods been affected today?

_____

_____

_____

_____

_____

_____

_____

_____

What foods and portion sizes have I eaten today?
How have my energy levels and moods been affected today?

_____

_____

_____

_____

_____

_____

day five

My dreams and plans are

week twelve

What exercises have I completed and for what duration?
How have my energy levels and moods been affected today?

_____

_____

_____

_____

_____

_____

_____

_____

What foods and portion sizes have I eaten today?
How have my energy levels and moods been affected today?

_____

_____

_____

_____

_____

_____

day six

Today I made someone happy because _____

week twelve

What exercises have I completed and for what duration?
How have my energy levels and moods been affected today?

What foods and portion sizes have I eaten today?
How have my energy levels and moods been affected today?

----

day seven

I will change the world by

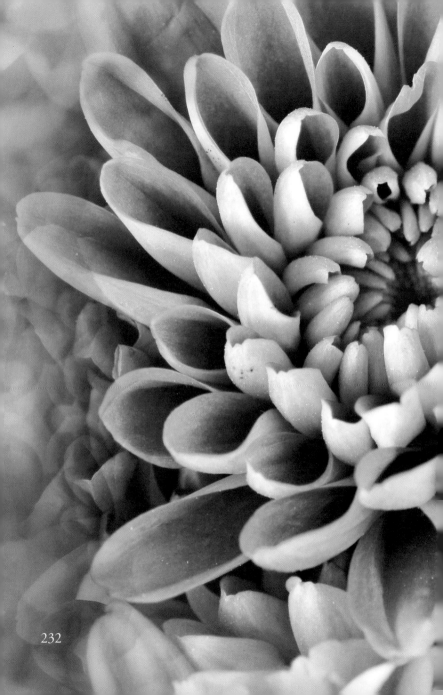

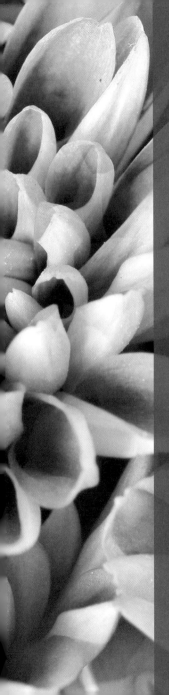

this is the beginning

It is now time to sit back and reflect on your personal growth and development over the last 12 weeks. Take the opportunity to review your goals that you set at the start of the journal and begin to soak up the change that has occurred for you physically, mentally, emotionally and spiritually.

Acknowledge the highs and lows of your journey and be proud of your persistence finishing what you started. Just the ability to complete what you started shows character that will serve you well through life. Now it's time to take this new insight into your life and inspire others by leading through example.

233

Write the biggest challenges you have conquered over the last 12 weeks:

_____

_____

_____

_____

_____

_____

_____

_____

_____

_____

_____

_____

_____

_____

_____

_____

_____

_____

_____

_____

_____

Write your new Goals:

235

Michelle Merrifield is the founder and operator of popular Essence of Living Yoga & Pilates studio and International Teacher Training Academy on the Gold Coast, Australia. After first discovering Yoga and Pilates at the young age of 16, Michelle knew this was her calling and she wanted to share both the spiritual and physical benefits of the practice with others.

To follow Michelle on her personal journey of discovery and transformation, follow her on Facebook:

Body Buddhaful | Facebook
www.facebook.com/pages/Body-Buddhaful

Michelle Merrifield | Facebook
www.facebook.com/michelle.merrifield.3

Essence of Living | Facebook
www.facebook.com/essenceofliving

"I live and breathe my vocation as it resonates with every cell of my body. I truly love what I do and do what I love. I want to share my passion with the world around me and hope to create a happier, healthier world with those willing to change and grow with me."

~ Michelle Merrifield